KIDNEY DISEASE DIET FOR SENIORS ON STAGE 3

A Comprehensive Guide To Thriving With Renal Disease Through Flavorful and Nourishing Low Sodium, Low Potassium and Low Phosphorus Kidney-friendly Recipes.

Joshua S. Gray

Copyright @ Joshua S. Gray 2023.
All rights reserved.
Before this document is duplicated or reproduced in any manner. The publisher's consent must be gained.
Therefore, the contents within can neither be stored electronically, transferred, nor kept in a database. Neither in part nor full can the document be copied, scanned, faxed or retained without approval from the publisher or creator.

For more information or help feel free to contact me at:

joshuagrayhelpdesk@gmail.com

Table of Contents

INTRODUCTION 7
CHAPTER 1 10
   What is Kidney Disease ? 10
   Potassium, Sodium, and Phosphorus in Managing kidney Disease 14
   Managing Electrolyte Levels in Kidney Disease: 17
CHAPTER 2 19
   Benefits of Kidney Diet 19
   Shopping List 24
CHAPTER 3 29
Breakfast Recipes 29
   1. Raspberry Peach Breakfast Smoothie 29
   2. Egg and Veggie Muffin 31
   3. Raspberry Overnight Porridge 33
   4. Spicy Corn Bread 35
   5. Summer Veggie Omelet 37
   6. Corn Bread with Southern Twist 39
   7. Breakfast Maple Sausage 41
   8. American Blueberry Pancakes 42
   9. Feta Mint Omelet 44
   10. Sausage Cheese Bake Omelet 46
CHAPTER 4 48
Fish and Seafood Recipes 48
   1. Haddock and Oiled Leeks 48
   2. Saucy Fish Dill 50
   3. Spanish Cod in Sauce 52

    4. Oregon Tuna Patties................................... 54
    5. Chili Mussels... 56
    6. Broiled Salmon Fillets............................... 58
    7. Fish Chili with Lentils.................................60
    8. Herbed Vegetable Trout........................... 62
    9. Tuna Casserole... 64
    10. Spiced Honey Salmon............................. 66

CHAPTER 5...**68**
Soup Recipes.. **68**
    1. Nutmeg and Chicken Soup........................ 68
    2. Squash and Turmeric Soup....................... 70
    3. Cabbage Turkey Soup.............................. 72
    4. Classic Chicken Soup............................... 74
    5. Mediterranean Vegetable Soup.................. 76
    6. Oxtail Soup...78
    7. Turkey and Lemongrass Soup................... 80
    8. Eggplant and Red Pepper Soup................ 82
    9. Chicken Wild Rice Soup............................84
    10. Beef Okra Soup..................................... 86

CHAPTER 6...**88**
Snack Recipes...**88**
    1. Marinated Berries......................................88
    2. Veggie Snack... 90
    3. Spicy Crab Dip... 91
    4. Sweet and Spicy Tortilla Chips...................93
    5. Buffalo Chicken Dip..................................95
    6. Mango Chiller... 96
    7. Vegetable Rolls.. 97
    8. Pecan Caramel Corn.................................99

- 9. Blueberry Ricotta Swirl..............................100
- 10. Spicy Guacamole....................................101

CHAPTER 7..**103**
Dessert Recipes..**103**
- 1. Chocolate Beet Cake............................... 103
- 2. Chocolate Muffins................................... 106
- 3. Pineapple Cake.......................................108
- 4. Strawberry Pie..110
- 5. Sweet Raspberry Candy......................... 112
- 6. Jeweled Cookies..................................... 114
- 7. Frozen Lemon Dessert............................116
- 8. Lemon Cake.. 118
- 9. Ribbon Cake... 120
- 10. Baked Egg Custard...............................122

30 Day Meal Plan..**124**
- Week 1.. 124
- Week 2.. 127
- Week 3.. 130
- Week 4.. 133

CONCLUSION...**137**
BONUS: WEEKLY MEAL PLANNER JOURNAL....140

TO GAIN ACCESS TO MORE BOOKS BY THE AUTHOR, SCAN THIS CODE

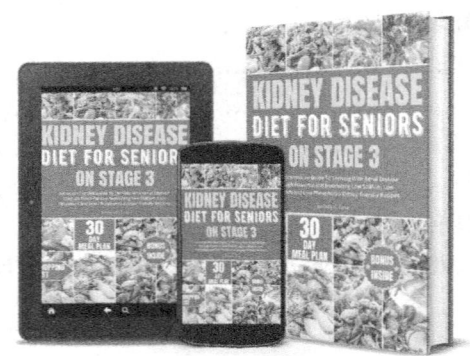

INTRODUCTION

Have you ever wondered what the best course of action is for managing Stage 3 kidney disease as a senior? The abundance of well-intended advice can be overwhelming, leaving many people with confusing ideas about what makes a healthy diet. There is a widespread belief that a restricted and flavorless diet is the key to treating renal diseases, but let me assure you that this thought is not only deceptive, but it can also deny you of the delight that a well-balanced and tasty meal can bring.

Making informed dietary decisions is essential for kidney disease, particularly when it is in its Stage 3 manifestation. Limitations are important, but so is designing a lifestyle that fits your particular health requirements and still lets you enjoy the tastes that make every meal a pleasure. Imagine a world in which taking care of your kidneys becomes a routine part of your day, and your plate is a source of nourishment and vigor rather than tension.

Within the pages of "Kidney Disease Diet For Seniors on Stage 3," we set out on an adventure that goes beyond conventional knowledge. This book is a thorough guide that takes into account your unique preferences, individuality, and desire for culinary satisfaction. It is not just a list of nutritional recommendations. What if you saw your condition as a chance to discover a world of delicious and nutritious meals catered to your unique needs, rather than as a set of limitations?

I understand the difficulties you are facing, the lingering doubts, and your desire for a remedy that improves your general health in addition to addressing the symptoms. This book is your companion to a happier, healthier life.

You'll find a lot of information in these pages, including tasty recipes, a well crafted meal plan, a road map for handling your Stage 3 kidney disease with assurance and clarity and lots more. Allow this book to serve as your ultimate source of empowerment and the answer to any unanswered questions that have been keeping you up at night.

Your well-being is my primary concern, and I encourage you to discover the life-changing opportunities that lie ahead in the upcoming chapters.

CHAPTER 1

What is Kidney Disease ?

Kidney disease, also known as renal disease, refers to a condition where the kidneys are damaged and unable to perform their normal functions adequately. The kidneys play a crucial role in maintaining overall health by filtering waste products and excess fluids from the blood, regulating electrolyte balance, and producing hormones that help control blood pressure and stimulate red blood cell production.

There are different types and stages of kidney disease, and they can be caused by various factors, including:

1. Diabetes: High levels of blood sugar can damage the blood vessels in the kidneys over time.
2. Hypertension (High Blood Pressure): Chronic high blood pressure can strain the blood vessels in the kidneys, leading to damage.
3. Genetic Factors: Some forms of kidney disease have a genetic component.
4. Infections: Certain infections can directly affect the kidneys.
5. Autoimmune Diseases: Conditions where the immune system attacks the body's own tissues can impact the kidneys.
6. Medications: Prolonged use of certain medications, like nonsteroidal

anti-inflammatory drugs (NSAIDs), can contribute to kidney damage.

Kidney disease may progress through various stages, typically categorized from Stage 1 to Stage 5, with Stage 5 being end-stage renal disease (ESRD). The severity of the disease and its progression depend on factors such as the underlying cause, lifestyle, and timely medical intervention.

Common symptoms of kidney disease may include fatigue, swelling, changes in urine output, and difficulty concentrating. Early detection and management are crucial to slowing the progression of kidney disease and preserving kidney function.

Treatment approaches may include lifestyle modifications, medications, and, in severe cases, dialysis or kidney transplantation.

Regular monitoring and collaboration with healthcare professionals are essential for managing kidney disease effectively.

Potassium, Sodium, and Phosphorus in Managing kidney Disease

Potassium, sodium, and phosphorus are electrolytes that play crucial roles in the body's normal functioning, and their levels are particularly important in managing kidney disease. Here's why each of these electrolytes is critical in the context of kidney health:

1. Potassium:
-   Normal Function: Potassium is essential for maintaining proper heart and muscle function, supporting the balance of fluids, and aiding in nerve signals.
-   Kidney Disease Impact: In advanced stages of kidney disease, the kidneys may struggle to regulate potassium levels. High

potassium levels (hyperkalemia) can pose a serious risk, leading to irregular heartbeats and other cardiovascular complications.

2. Sodium:

- Normal Function: Sodium is essential for maintaining proper fluid balance, supporting nerve function, and aiding in muscle contraction.

- Kidney Disease Impact: Kidneys affected by kidney disease may have difficulty excreting excess sodium, leading to sodium retention. High sodium levels (hypernatremia) can contribute to fluid retention, swelling, and increased blood pressure, which can further strain the kidneys.

3. **Phosphorus:**

- Normal Function: Phosphorus is crucial for bone health, energy production, and various cellular functions.

- Kidney Disease Impact: In kidney disease, the kidneys may struggle to excrete excess phosphorus, leading to elevated phosphorus levels (hyperphosphatemia). High phosphorus levels can contribute to mineral and bone disorders, leading to weakened bones and cardiovascular complications.

Managing Electrolyte Levels in Kidney Disease:

- **Dietary Restrictions:** Controlling the intake of potassium, sodium, and phosphorus through dietary restrictions is a common strategy. This involves avoiding high-potassium foods (e.g., bananas, oranges), limiting sodium intake, and monitoring phosphorus-rich foods (e.g., dairy products, nuts).

- **Medications:** Phosphate binders may be prescribed to help control phosphorus levels by binding to phosphorus in the digestive tract and preventing its absorption.

- **Fluid Management:** Maintaining proper fluid balance is crucial in managing sodium levels. In some cases, fluid intake may be restricted to prevent fluid retention.

Monitoring and managing these electrolyte levels are integral parts of a comprehensive approach to kidney disease management. Regular check-ups, blood tests, and collaboration with healthcare professionals, including dietitians, are essential to tailor interventions based on individual needs and the stage of kidney disease.

CHAPTER 2

Benefits of Kidney Diet

A kidney-friendly diet, tailored to the specific needs of individuals with kidney disease, offers numerous benefits that contribute to overall health and well-being. Here are some key benefits:

1. **Preservation of Kidney Function:** A kidney diet aims to manage the intake of certain nutrients, such as sodium, potassium, and phosphorus, which can help slow the progression of kidney disease and preserve remaining kidney function.

2. **Blood Pressure Control:** Sodium restriction is a crucial aspect of a kidney diet. By reducing sodium intake, blood pressure can

be better controlled, which is essential for kidney health.

3. **Electrolyte Balance:** Managing potassium and phosphorus levels is critical. A kidney diet helps prevent imbalances in these electrolytes, which can otherwise lead to complications such as irregular heartbeats and bone disorders.

4. **Heart Health:** Many aspects of a kidney diet, including reduced sodium intake and control of certain minerals, contribute to improved cardiovascular health. This is particularly important, as individuals with kidney disease often have an increased risk of heart-related complications.

5. **Prevention of Complications:** By controlling the intake of certain nutrients, a kidney diet helps prevent complications

associated with kidney disease, such as fluid retention, swelling, and mineral and bone disorders.

6. **Management of Symptoms:** Following a kidney diet can alleviate symptoms associated with kidney disease, such as fatigue, nausea, and changes in urine output.

7. **Customization for Individual Needs:** A kidney diet is not a one-size-fits-all approach. It can be customized based on the individual's stage of kidney disease, specific nutrient needs, and personal preferences. This customization ensures that dietary recommendations align with the unique requirements of each person.

8. **Improved Quality of Life:** By addressing nutritional needs and minimizing complications, a kidney diet contributes to an improved quality of life for individuals with

kidney disease. It allows for a more thoughtful and enjoyable approach to food while promoting overall health.

9. **Nutritional Support:** A kidney diet is designed to provide adequate nutrition while managing specific dietary restrictions. It ensures that individuals receive essential nutrients, vitamins, and minerals necessary for overall well-being.

10. **Collaboration with Healthcare Professionals:** Following a kidney diet involves collaboration with healthcare professionals, including dietitians and nephrologists. This ongoing support and guidance contribute to a more comprehensive and effective management approach.

It's important to note that the benefits of a kidney diet may vary based on individual health conditions, the stage of kidney disease, and other factors. Individuals with kidney disease should work closely with their healthcare team to develop a personalized dietary plan that addresses their specific needs and goals.

Shopping List

When preparing a shopping list for a kidney disease diet for seniors in Stage 3, it's essential to focus on foods that help manage sodium, potassium, and phosphorus levels. Here's a general shopping list to guide you:

Protein Sources:
1. Skinless poultry (chicken or turkey)
2. Lean cuts of beef or pork
3. Fish (low in phosphorus, such as salmon, trout, or tilapia)
4. Eggs
5. Cottage cheese
6. Tofu

Fruits:

7. Apples
8. Berries (strawberries, blueberries, raspberries)
9. Pineapple
10. Watermelon
11. Grapes
12. Cranberries (as juice or fresh)

Vegetables:

13. Bell peppers
14. Cabbage
15. Cauliflower
16. Broccoli
17. Carrots
18. Zucchini
19. Onion
20. Garlic

Grains and Starches:

21. White rice
22. White bread
23. Pasta
24. Cornflakes or rice cereals (low in phosphorus)
25. Oatmeal (limit portion size)

Dairy and Dairy Alternatives:

26. Low-fat or fat-free milk
27. Low-fat or fat-free yogurt
28. Almond milk or rice milk (low in phosphorus)

Snacks:

29. Rice cakes
30. Popcorn (limit butter and salt)
31. Unsalted crackers
32. Hard candy or popsicles (for dry mouth)

Beverages:

33. Water (main hydration source)

34. Herbal teas (avoid those with hibiscus)

35. Lemonade (homemade with controlled sugar)

Herbs and Spices:

36. Fresh herbs (parsley, cilantro, basil)

37. Dried spices (avoid seasoning blends with added salt)

38. Lemon or lime juice

Fats and Oils:

39. Olive oil

40. Canola oil

Sweeteners:

41. Honey

42. Maple syrup

Avoid or Limit:

- High-potassium fruits (bananas, oranges, melons)
- High-potassium vegetables (potatoes, tomatoes)
- High-phosphorus foods (dairy, nuts, seeds)
- Processed and salty foods (canned soups, processed meats)
- Dark colas and sodas
- High-sodium condiments (soy sauce, ketchup)

CHAPTER 3

Breakfast Recipes

1. Raspberry Peach Breakfast Smoothie

Ingredients:
- ½ cup raspberries
- ½ cup sliced peaches
- ½ cup low-fat or almond milk
- ½ cup Greek yogurt (low potassium)
- Ice cubes (optional)

Preparation:
1. Blend all ingredients until smooth.
2. Add ice cubes if desired.
3. Serve immediately.

Nutritional Information:

- Calories: 150
- Protein: 8g
- Carbohydrates: 25g
- Fiber: 5g
- Potassium: 200mg

2. Egg and Veggie Muffin

Ingredients:

- 2 eggs
- ¼ cup diced bell peppers
- ¼ cup diced tomatoes
- 2 tablespoons diced onions
- Salt and pepper to taste

Preparation:

1. Preheat oven to 350°F (175°C).
2. Whisk eggs and season with pepper and salt.
3. Stir in diced vegetables.
4. Pour into muffin cups.
5. Bake for 15-20 minutes or until eggs are set.

Nutritional Information:
- Calories: 150
- Protein: 12g
- Carbohydrates: 5g
- Fiber: 1g
- Potassium: 170mg

3. Raspberry Overnight Porridge

Ingredients:

- ½ cup rolled oats
- ½ cup of almond milk
- ¼ cup raspberries
- 1 tablespoon chia seeds
- 1 tablespoon honey

Preparation:

1. Mix oats, milk, raspberries, and chia seeds in a jar.
2. Refrigerate overnight.
3. In the morning, drizzle with honey before serving.

Nutritional Information:

- Calories: 250
- Protein: 8g
- Carbohydrates: 40g
- Fiber: 8g
- Potassium: 180mg

4. Spicy Corn Bread

Ingredients:

- 1 cup cornmeal
- ½ cup whole wheat flour
- 1 tablespoon baking powder
- ½ teaspoon salt
- ½ teaspoon chili powder
- 1 cup low-fat buttermilk
- ¼ cup canola oil
- 2 eggs

Preparation:

1. Preheat oven to 400°F (200°C).
2. Mix dry ingredients in one bowl, wet ingredients in another, then combine.
3. Pour into a greased baking dish.
4. Bake for 20-25 minutes or until a toothpick comes out clean.

Nutritional Information:

- Calories: 150
- Protein: 5g
- Carbohydrates: 20g
- Fiber: 2g
- Potassium: 90mg

5. Summer Veggie Omelet

Ingredients:

- 2 eggs
- ¼ cup diced zucchini
- ¼ cup diced tomatoes
- 2 tablespoons diced red bell peppers
- 1 tablespoon chopped fresh basil
- Salt and pepper to taste

Preparation:

1. Whisk eggs and season with pepper and salt.
2. Pour into a heated, greased skillet.
3. Sprinkle vegetables and basil over half of the eggs.
4. Fold the other half over the veggies.
5. Cook until eggs are set.

Nutritional Information:

- Calories: 180
- Protein: 12g
- Carbohydrates: 5g
- Fiber: 1g
- Potassium: 220mg

6. Corn Bread with Southern Twist

Ingredients:

- 1 cup cornmeal
- ½ cup whole wheat flour
- 1 tablespoon baking powder
- ½ teaspoon salt
- ¼ cup unsweetened applesauce
- ¼ cup canola oil
- 2/3 cup low-fat milk

Preparation:

1. Preheat oven to 400°F (200°C).
2. Mix dry ingredients in one bowl, wet ingredients in another, then combine.
3. Pour into a greased baking dish.
4. Bake for 20-25 minutes or until a toothpick comes out clean.

Nutritional Information:
- Calories: 160
- Protein: 4g
- Carbohydrates: 22g
- Fiber: 2g
- Potassium: 80mg

7. Breakfast Maple Sausage

Ingredients:

- 4 lean turkey or chicken sausage links
- 1 tablespoon maple syrup (low potassium)

Preparation:

1. Cook sausage links according to package instructions.
2. Drizzle with maple syrup before serving.

Nutritional Information:

- Calories: 200
- Protein: 12g
- Carbohydrates: 5g
- Fiber: 0g
- Potassium: 180mg

8. American Blueberry Pancakes

Ingredients:

- 1 cup whole wheat flour
- 1 tablespoon baking powder
- ½ teaspoon salt
- 1 cup low-fat milk
- 1 egg
- 1 cup fresh blueberries

Preparation:

1. Mix dry ingredients, then add wet ingredients.
2. Fold in blueberries.
3. Cook on a griddle until bubbles form, then flip.

Nutritional Information:

- Calories: 180
- Protein: 7g
- Carbohydrates: 35g
- Fiber: 5g
- Potassium: 220mg

9. Feta Mint Omelet

Ingredients:

- 2 eggs
- 2 tablespoons crumbled feta cheese
- 1 tablespoon chopped fresh mint
- Salt and pepper to taste

Preparation:

1. Whisk eggs and season with pepper and salt.
2. Pour into a heated, greased skillet.
3. Sprinkle feta and mint over half of the eggs.
4. Over the filling, fold the other half.
5. Cook until eggs are set.

Nutritional Information:

- Calories: 200
- Protein: 12g
- Carbohydrates: 2g
- Fiber: 0g
- Potassium: 220mg

10. Sausage Cheese Bake Omelet

Ingredients:

- 2 eggs
- 2 lean turkey or chicken sausage links, cooked and diced
- 2 tablespoons shredded low-fat cheddar cheese
- Salt and pepper to taste

Preparation:

1. Whisk eggs and season with pepper and salt.
2. Pour into a heated, greased skillet.
3. Sprinkle cooked sausage and cheese over half of the eggs.
4. Over the filling, fold the other half.
5. Cook until eggs are set.

Nutritional Information:
- Calories: 250
- Protein: 15g
- Carbohydrates: 3g
- Fiber: 0g
- Potassium: 180mg

CHAPTER 4

Fish and Seafood Recipes

1. Haddock and Oiled Leeks

Ingredients:

- 2 haddock fillets
- 1 leek, thinly sliced
- Olive oil
- Salt and pepper to taste

Preparation:

1. Preheat oven to 375°F (190°C).
2. Place haddock fillets on a baking dish.
3. Scatter sliced leeks over the fillets.
4. Drizzle with olive oil, season with salt and pepper to make it more appetising.

5. Bake for 15-20 minutes or until fish is cooked.

Nutritional Information:
- Calories: 180
- Protein: 25g
- Carbohydrates: 3g
- Fiber: 1g
- Potassium: 350mg

2. Saucy Fish Dill

Ingredients:

- 2 white fish fillets
- ¼ cup low-sodium chicken broth
- 1 tablespoon fresh dill, chopped
- Lemon juice
- Salt and pepper to taste

Preparation:

1. In a skillet, combine dill, lemon juice, pepper, broth, and salt.
2. Place fish fillets in the skillet.
3. Simmer for 10-15 minutes or until fish is cooked.

Nutritional Information:

- Calories: 160
- Protein: 20g
- Carbohydrates: 1g
- Fiber: 0g
- Potassium: 280mg

3. Spanish Cod in Sauce

Ingredients:

- 2 cod fillets
- 1 cup tomato sauce (low sodium)
- ¼ cup green olives, sliced
- ¼ teaspoon paprika
- Salt and pepper to taste

Preparation:

1. Preheat oven to 375°F (190°C).
2. Place cod fillets in a baking dish.
3. Mix tomato sauce, olives, paprika, salt, and pepper.
4. Pour the sauce over the cod.
5. Bake for 20-25 minutes or until fish is done.

Nutritional Information:

- Calories: 190
- Protein: 25g
- Carbohydrates: 5g
- Fiber: 2g
- Potassium: 400mg

4. Oregon Tuna Patties

Ingredients:

- 1 can tuna, drained
- ¼ cup whole wheat breadcrumbs
- 1 egg
- 2 tablespoons fresh parsley, chopped
- Lemon wedges

Preparation:

1. Mix tuna, breadcrumbs, egg, and parsley.
2. Form into patties.
3. Cook in a skillet until golden brown.
4. Serve with lemon wedges.

Nutritional Information:

- Calories: 160
- Protein: 20g
- Carbohydrates: 5g
- Fiber: 1g
- Potassium: 220mg

5. Chili Mussels

Ingredients:

- 1 pound mussels, cleaned
- 1 cup low-sodium chicken broth
- ½ cup diced tomatoes
- ¼ cup chopped cilantro
- 1 teaspoon chili powder

Preparation:

1. In a pot, combine broth, tomatoes, cilantro, and chili powder.
2. Bring to a simmer.
3. Add mussels and cook until they open.
4. Discard any unopened mussels.

Nutritional Information:

- Calories: 180
- Protein: 20g
- Carbohydrates: 7g
- Fiber: 1g
- Potassium: 350mg

6. Broiled Salmon Fillets

Ingredients:

- 2 salmon fillets
- 1 tablespoon olive oil
- Lemon slices
- Fresh herbs (thyme, rosemary)
- Salt and pepper to taste

Preparation:

1. Preheat broiler.
2. Brush salmon with olive oil.
3. Season with salt, pepper, and herbs.
4. Broil for 10-15 minutes or until salmon is cooked.
5. Serve with lemon slices.

Nutritional Information:

- Calories: 220
- Protein: 25g
- Carbohydrates: 0g
- Fiber: 0g
- Potassium: 350mg

7. Fish Chili with Lentils

Ingredients:

- 1 cup cooked lentils
- 1 white fish fillet, flaked
- 1 cup tomato sauce (low sodium)
- ½ cup diced bell peppers
- ½ teaspoon cumin
- Salt and pepper to taste

Preparation:

1. In a pot, combine lentils, fish, tomato sauce, peppers, cumin, salt, and pepper.
2. Simmer for 15-20 minutes.

Nutritional Information:

- Calories: 240
- Protein: 20g
- Carbohydrates: 30g
- Fiber: 9g
- Potassium: 450mg

8. Herbed Vegetable Trout

Ingredients:

- 2 trout fillets
- ½ cup cherry tomatoes, halved
- ¼ cup sliced zucchini
- 1 tablespoon olive oil
- Fresh herbs (parsley, dill)
- Salt and pepper to taste

Preparation:

1. Preheat oven to 375°F (190°C).
2. Place trout fillets on a baking sheet.
3. Scatter tomatoes and zucchini around the fish.
4. Drizzle with olive oil, sprinkle with herbs, salt, and pepper.
5. Bake for 15-20 minutes or until fish is done.

Nutritional Information:

- Calories: 210
- Protein: 25g
- Carbohydrates: 5g
- Fiber: 2g
- Potassium: 320mg

9. Tuna Casserole

Ingredients:

- 2 cups cooked whole wheat pasta
- 1 can tuna, drained
- 1 cup frozen peas
- ½ cup low-fat milk
- 2 tablespoons whole wheat flour
- ¼ cup shredded low-fat cheddar cheese

Preparation:

1. Mix pasta, tuna, and peas in a baking dish.
2. In a saucepan, whisk milk, flour, and cheese until smooth.
3. Pour over the pasta mixture.
4. Bake at 350°F (175°C) for 20 minutes.

Nutritional Information:

- Calories: 260
- Protein: 20g
- Carbohydrates: 30g
- Fiber: 5g
- Potassium: 300mg

10. Spiced Honey Salmon

Ingredients:

- 2 salmon fillets
- 2 tablespoons honey
- 1 teaspoon paprika
- ½ teaspoon cayenne pepper
- Salt and pepper to taste

Preparation:

1. Preheat oven to 375°F (190°C).
2. Mix honey, paprika, cayenne, salt, and pepper.
3. Brush the mixture over salmon.
4. Bake for 15-20 minutes or until salmon is cooked.

Nutritional Information:
- Calories: 230
- Protein: 25g
- Carbohydrates: 10g
- Fiber: 1g
- Potassium: 300mg

CHAPTER 5

Soup Recipes

1. Nutmeg and Chicken Soup

Ingredients:

- 1 cup cooked chicken, shredded
- 4 cups low-sodium chicken broth
- ½ teaspoon nutmeg
- ½ cup carrots, diced
- ½ cup celery, diced
- Salt and pepper to taste

Preparation:

1. In a pot, combine chicken, chicken broth, nutmeg, carrots, and celery.
2. Simmer for 15-20 minutes.
3. Season with salt and pepper.

Nutritional Information:

- Calories: 150
- Protein: 20g
- Carbohydrates: 5g
- Fiber: 1g
- Potassium: 300mg

2. Squash and Turmeric Soup

Ingredients:

- 2 cups of butternut squash, peeled and diced
- 4 cups low-sodium vegetable broth
- 1 teaspoon turmeric
- ½ cup onion, chopped
- ½ cup coconut milk
- Salt and pepper to taste

Preparation:

1. In a pot, combine squash, vegetable broth, turmeric, and onion.
2. Simmer until squash is tender.
3. Blend until smooth.
4. Stir in coconut milk.
5. Season with salt and pepper.

Nutritional Information:

- Calories: 120
- Protein: 2g
- Carbohydrates: 20g
- Fiber: 3g
- Potassium: 450mg

3. Cabbage Turkey Soup

Ingredients:

- 1 cup cooked turkey, diced
- 4 cups low-sodium chicken broth
- 2 cups cabbage, shredded
- ½ cup carrots, sliced
- ½ cup onion, diced
- 1 teaspoon thyme
- Salt and pepper to taste

Preparation:

1. In a pot, combine turkey, chicken broth, cabbage, carrots, onion, and thyme.
2. Simmer for 20-25 minutes.
3. Season with salt and pepper.

Nutritional Information:
- Calories: 180
- Protein: 15g
- Carbohydrates: 10g
- Fiber: 4g
- Potassium: 320mg

4. Classic Chicken Soup

Ingredients:

- 1 cup cooked chicken, shredded
- 4 cups low-sodium chicken broth
- ½ cup carrots, diced
- ½ cup celery, diced
- ½ cup noodles (low-phosphorus)
- 1 teaspoon parsley
- Salt and pepper to taste

Preparation:

1. In a pot, combine chicken, chicken broth, carrots, celery, and noodles.
2. Simmer until vegetables are tender.
3. Stir in parsley.
4. Season with salt and pepper.

Nutritional Information:

- Calories: 200
- Protein: 20g
- Carbohydrates: 15g
- Fiber: 2g
- Potassium: 300mg

5. Mediterranean Vegetable Soup

Ingredients:
- 4 cups low-sodium vegetable broth
- 1 cup zucchini, diced
- 1 cup bell peppers, diced
- ½ cup tomatoes, diced
- ½ cup chickpeas, cooked
- 1 teaspoon oregano
- Salt and pepper to taste

Preparation:
1. In a pot, combine vegetable broth, zucchini, bell peppers, tomatoes, chickpeas, and oregano.
2. Simmer for 15-20 minutes.
3. Season with salt and pepper.

Nutritional Information:

- Calories: 120
- Protein: 5g
- Carbohydrates: 20g
- Fiber: 5g
- Potassium: 450mg

6. Oxtail Soup

Ingredients:

- 2 lbs oxtail, trimmed
- 6 cups water
- ½ cup carrots, sliced
- ½ cup celery, sliced
- ½ cup onion, diced
- 2 cloves garlic, minced
- 1 bay leaf
- Salt and pepper to taste

Preparation:

1. In a large pot, combine oxtail, water, carrots, celery, onion, garlic, and bay leaf.
2. Boil and simmer for 2-3 hours until oxtail is tender.
3. Season with salt and pepper.

Nutritional Information:

- Calories: 250
- Protein: 25g
- Carbohydrates: 5g
- Fiber: 1g
- Potassium: 350mg

7. Turkey and Lemongrass Soup

Ingredients:

- 1 cup cooked turkey, shredded
- 4 cups low-sodium chicken broth
- 1 stalk lemongrass, sliced
- ½ cup mushrooms, sliced
- ½ cup bok choy, chopped
- 1 teaspoon ginger, minced
- Salt and pepper to taste

Preparation:

1. In a pot, combine turkey, chicken broth, lemongrass, mushrooms, bok choy, and ginger.
2. Simmer for 15-20 minutes.
3. Season with salt and pepper.

Nutritional Information:
- Calories: 150
- Protein: 15g
- Carbohydrates: 5g
- Fiber: 2g
- Potassium: 300mg

8. Eggplant and Red Pepper Soup

Ingredients:

- 2 cups eggplant, diced
- 4 cups low-sodium vegetable broth
- 1 cup red bell pepper, diced
- ½ cup onion, diced
- 2 cloves garlic, minced
- 1 teaspoon cumin
- Salt and pepper to taste

Preparation:

1. In a pot, combine eggplant, vegetable broth, red bell pepper, onion, garlic, and cumin.
2. Simmer until vegetables are tender.
3. Season with salt and pepper.

Nutritional Information:

- Calories: 130
- Protein: 3g
- Carbohydrates: 25g
- Fiber: 6g
- Potassium: 450mg

9. Chicken Wild Rice Soup

Ingredients:

- 1 cup cooked chicken, shredded
- 4 cups low-sodium chicken broth
- ½ cup wild rice, cooked
- ½ cup carrots, diced
- ½ cup celery, diced
- ½ cup mushrooms, sliced
- 1 teaspoon thyme
- Salt and pepper to taste

Preparation:

1. In a pot, combine chicken, chicken broth, wild rice, carrots, celery, mushrooms, and thyme.
2. Simmer for 20-25 minutes.
3. Season with salt and pepper.

Nutritional Information:

- Calories: 180
- Protein: 15g
- Carbohydrates: 20g
- Fiber: 3g
- Potassium: 320mg

10. Beef Okra Soup

Ingredients:

- ½ lb lean beef, diced
- 4 cups water
- 1 cup okra, sliced
- ½ cup tomatoes, diced
- ½ cup onion, diced
- ½ cup carrots, sliced
- ½ cup celery, sliced
- 1 teaspoon thyme
- Salt and pepper to taste

Preparation:

1. In a pot, combine beef, water, okra, tomatoes, onion, carrots, celery, thyme, salt, and pepper.
2. Boil and simmer for 30-40 minutes.

Nutritional Information:

- Calories: 200
- Protein: 20g
- Carbohydrates: 10g
- Fiber: 3g
- Potassium: 350mg

CHAPTER 6

Snack Recipes

1. Marinated Berries

Ingredients:

- 1 cup mixed strawberries, blueberries, raspberries
- 1 tablespoon balsamic vinegar
- 1 teaspoon honey
- Fresh mint leaves for garnish

Preparation:

1. In a bowl, mix berries, balsamic vinegar, and honey.
2. Let it marinate in the refrigerator for at least 30 minutes.
3. Garnish with fresh mint before serving.

Nutritional Information:

- Calories: 50
- Protein: 1g
- Carbohydrates: 12g
- Fiber: 3g
- Potassium: 150mg

2. Veggie Snack

Ingredients:
- 1 cup cucumber, sliced
- 1 cup cherry tomatoes, halved
- ½ cup carrot sticks
- ¼ cup hummus for dipping

Preparation:
1. Arrange cucumber, cherry tomatoes, and carrot sticks on a plate.
2. Serve with hummus for dipping.

Nutritional Information:
- Calories: 80
- Protein: 3g
- Carbohydrates: 15g
- Fiber: 4g
- Potassium: 300mg

3. Spicy Crab Dip

Ingredients:

- 1 cup lump crab meat
- ½ cup Greek yogurt
- 1 tablespoon hot sauce
- 1 teaspoon lemon juice
- ¼ teaspoon Old Bay seasoning
- Chopped chives for garnish

Preparation:

1. In a bowl, mix crab meat, Greek yogurt, hot sauce, lemon juice, and Old Bay seasoning.
2. Garnish with chopped chives before serving.

Nutritional Information:
- Calories: 90
- Protein: 15g
- Carbohydrates: 3g
- Fiber: 0g
- Potassium: 200mg

4. Sweet and Spicy Tortilla Chips

Ingredients:

- 4 whole-grain tortillas
- 1 tablespoon olive oil
- 1 teaspoon cinnamon
- ½ teaspoon cayenne pepper
- 1 tablespoon honey

Preparation:

1. Preheat oven to 350°F (175°C).
2. Brush tortillas with olive oil.
3. Mix cinnamon and cayenne pepper; sprinkle over tortillas.
4. Cut into wedges and bake for 10 minutes.
5. Drizzle with honey.

Nutritional Information:

- Calories: 100
- Protein: 2g
- Carbohydrates: 15g
- Fiber: 2g
- Potassium: 120mg

5. Buffalo Chicken Dip

Ingredients:

- 1 cup shredded cooked chicken
- ½ cup Greek yogurt
- 2 tablespoons hot sauce
- ¼ cup crumbled blue cheese
- Celery sticks for dipping

Preparation:

1. In a bowl, mix shredded chicken, Greek yogurt, hot sauce, and blue cheese.
2. Serve with celery sticks for dipping.

Nutritional Information:

- Calories: 120
- Protein: 15g
- Carbohydrates: 3g
- Fiber: 0g
- Potassium: 200mg

6. Mango Chiller

Ingredients:
- 1 cup frozen mango chunks
- ½ cup coconut water
- ¼ cup fresh lime juice
- Ice cubes

Preparation:

1. Blend frozen mango chunks, coconut water, and lime juice until smooth.
2. Serve over ice.

Nutritional Information:
- Calories: 80
- Protein: 1g
- Carbohydrates: 20g
- Fiber: 2g
- Potassium: 200mg

7. Vegetable Rolls

Ingredients:

- Rice paper sheets
- Thinly sliced vegetables (carrots, cucumber, bell peppers)
- Fresh herbs (mint, cilantro)
- Dipping sauce (low-sodium soy sauce, lime juice)

Preparation:

1. Dip rice paper sheets in warm water to soften.
2. Fill with sliced vegetables and fresh herbs.
3. Roll tightly and serve with dipping sauce.

Nutritional Information:
- Calories: 70
- Protein: 2g
- Carbohydrates: 15g
- Fiber: 2g
- Potassium: 250mg

8. Pecan Caramel Corn

Ingredients:

- 4 cups air-popped popcorn
- ½ cup pecans, chopped
- 2 tablespoons caramel sauce

Preparation:

1. Mix air-popped popcorn and chopped pecans.
2. Drizzle with caramel sauce and toss to coat.

Nutritional Information:

- Calories: 120
- Protein: 2g
- Carbohydrates: 20g
- Fiber: 3g
- Potassium: 80mg

9. Blueberry Ricotta Swirl

Ingredients:

- ½ cup low-fat ricotta cheese
- ½ cup fresh blueberries
- 1 tablespoon honey

Preparation:

1. In a bowl, swirl together ricotta cheese and blueberries.
2. Drizzle with honey before serving.

Nutritional Information:

- Calories: 130
- Protein: 8g
- Carbohydrates: 15g
- Fiber: 2g
- Potassium: 180mg

10. Spicy Guacamole

Ingredients:

- 2 ripe avocados, mashed
- ½ cup tomatoes, diced
- ¼ cup red onion, finely chopped
- 1 jalapeño, minced
- 2 tablespoons fresh cilantro, chopped
- Salt and lime juice to taste

Preparation:

1. In a bowl, combine mashed avocados, tomatoes, red onion, jalapeño, and cilantro.
2. Season with salt and lime juice.

Nutritional Information:

- Calories: 100
- Protein: 2g
- Carbohydrates: 8g
- Fiber: 5g
- Potassium: 400mg

CHAPTER 7

Dessert Recipes

1. Chocolate Beet Cake

Ingredients:

- 2 cups cooked and pureed beets
- 1 ½ cups whole wheat flour
- ½ cup unsweetened cocoa powder
- 1 cup honey or maple syrup
- ½ cup Greek yogurt
- 2 eggs
- 1 teaspoon vanilla extract
- 1 ½ teaspoons baking powder
- ½ teaspoon baking soda
- ¼ teaspoon salt

Preparation:

1. Preheat oven to 350°F (175°C) and grease a cake pan.

2. In a bowl, mix together pureed beets, honey or maple syrup, Greek yogurt, eggs, and vanilla extract.

3. In another bowl, combine whole wheat flour, cocoa powder, baking powder, baking soda, and salt.

4. Add the dry ingredients to the wet components gradually and stir until thoroughly blended.

5. Pour the batter into the prepared cake pan and bake for 25-30 minutes or until a toothpick comes out clean.

Nutritional Information:

- Calories: 180
- Protein: 6g
- Carbohydrates: 38g
- Fiber: 6g
- Potassium: 250mg

2. Chocolate Muffins

Ingredients:

- 1 ½ cups almond flour
- ¼ cup unsweetened cocoa powder
- ½ teaspoon baking soda
- ¼ teaspoon salt
- 3 large eggs
- ¼ cup coconut oil, melted
- ¼ cup honey or maple syrup
- 1 teaspoon vanilla extract
- ½ cup dark chocolate chips (optional)

Preparation:

1. Preheat oven to 350°F (175°C) and line a muffin tin with paper liners.

2. In a bowl, whisk together almond flour, cocoa powder, baking soda, and salt.

3. In another bowl, beat the eggs and add melted coconut oil, honey or maple syrup, and vanilla extract.

4. Combine the wet and dry ingredients, mixing until just combined.

5. Fold in chocolate chips if desired.

6. Spoon the batter into the muffin cups and bake for 15-20 minutes.

Nutritional Information:

- Calories: 180
- Protein: 6g
- Carbohydrates: 15g
- Fiber: 3g
- Potassium: 200mg

3. Pineapple Cake

Ingredients:

- 2 cups crushed pineapple, drained
- 1 ½ cups almond flour
- ½ cup coconut flour
- 1 teaspoon baking soda
- ¼ teaspoon salt
- 3 large eggs
- ¼ cup coconut oil, melted
- ¼ cup honey or maple syrup
- 1 teaspoon vanilla extract

Preparation:

1. Preheat oven to 350°F (175°C) and grease a cake pan.
2. In a bowl, combine crushed pineapple, almond flour, coconut flour, baking soda, and salt.

3. In another bowl, beat the eggs and add melted coconut oil, honey or maple syrup, and vanilla extract.

4. Mix the wet and dry ingredients until well combined.

5. Pour the batter into the prepared cake pan and bake for 25-30 minutes.

Nutritional Information:
- Calories: 200
- Protein: 7g
- Carbohydrates: 18g
- Fiber: 4g
- Potassium: 180mg

4. Strawberry Pie

Ingredients:

- 2 cups fresh strawberries, sliced
- ¼ cup honey or maple syrup
- 1 tablespoon cornstarch
- 1 tablespoon lemon juice
- 1 pre-made whole wheat pie crust

Preparation:

1. In a saucepan, combine strawberries, honey or maple syrup, cornstarch, and lemon juice.
2. Cook over medium heat until the mixture thickens.
3. Allow the strawberry filling to cool.
4. Pour the cooled filling into the pre-made pie crust.

5. Before serving, let it cool in the fridge for a minimum of two hours.

Nutritional Information:
- Calories: 160
- Protein: 3g
- Carbohydrates: 30g
- Fiber: 4g
- Potassium: 200mg

5. Sweet Raspberry Candy

Ingredients:

- 1 cup fresh raspberries
- ¼ cup unsweetened shredded coconut
- 1 tablespoon honey or maple syrup

Preparation:

1. Dip each raspberry into honey or maple syrup.
2. Roll the coated raspberry in shredded coconut.
3. Transfer to a parchment paper-lined tray.
4. Chill in the refrigerator for 30 minutes before serving.

Nutritional Information:

- Calories: 60
- Protein: 1g
- Carbohydrates: 10g
- Fiber: 4g
- Potassium: 100mg

6. Jeweled Cookies

Ingredients:

- 1 ½ cups almond flour
- ¼ cup coconut flour
- ¼ cup coconut oil, melted
- ¼ cup honey or maple syrup
- 1 teaspoon vanilla extract
- ¼ cup mixed dried fruits (apricots, cranberries, raisins)

Preparation:

1. Adjust the oven temperature to 350°F (175°C) and place parchment paper on a baking pan.
2. In a bowl, combine almond flour, coconut flour, melted coconut oil, honey or maple syrup, and vanilla extract.
3. Fold in mixed dried fruits.

4. Form small cookies and place them on the prepared baking sheet.

5. Bake for 10-12 minutes or until the edges are golden brown.

Nutritional Information:
- Calories: 120
- Protein: 3g
- Carbohydrates: 10g
- Fiber: 2g
- Potassium: 150mg

7. Frozen Lemon Dessert

Ingredients:

- 2 cups Greek yogurt
- ¼ cup lemon juice
- ¼ cup honey or maple syrup
- 1 teaspoon lemon zest

Preparation:

1. In a bowl, mix together Greek yogurt, lemon juice, honey or maple syrup, and lemon zest.
2. Pour the mixture into a shallow dish and freeze for at least 4 hours.
3. Scoop and serve.

Nutritional Information:

- Calories: 150
- Protein: 8g
- Carbohydrates: 20g
- Fiber: 1g
- Potassium: 200mg

8. Lemon Cake

Ingredients:

- 2 cups almond flour
- ¼ cup coconut flour
- 1 teaspoon baking soda
- ¼ teaspoon salt
- 3 large eggs
- ¼ cup coconut oil, melted
- ¼ cup honey or maple syrup
- ¼ cup lemon juice
- 1 teaspoon lemon zest

Preparation:

1. Preheat oven to 350°F (175°C) and grease a cake pan.
2. In a bowl, whisk together baking soda, salt, almond flour, and coconut flour.

3. In another bowl, beat the eggs and add melted coconut oil, honey or maple syrup, lemon juice, and lemon zest.

4. Combine the wet and dry ingredients, mixing until just combined.

5. Pour the batter into the prepared cake pan and bake for 25-30 minutes.

Nutritional Information:
- Calories: 190
- Protein: 6g
- Carbohydrates: 15g
- Fiber: 3g
- Potassium: 180mg

9. Ribbon Cake

Ingredients:

- 2 cups almond flour
- ¼ cup coconut flour
- 1 teaspoon baking soda
- ¼ teaspoon salt
- 3 large eggs
- ¼ cup coconut oil, melted
- ¼ cup honey or maple syrup
- 1 teaspoon vanilla extract
- ¼ cup dark chocolate chips

Preparation:

1. Preheat oven to 350°F (175°C) and grease a loaf pan.
2. In a bowl, whisk together baking soda, salt, almond flour, and coconut flour.

3. In another bowl, beat the eggs and add melted coconut oil, honey or maple syrup, and vanilla extract.

4. Mix the wet and dry ingredients until well combined.

5. Fold in dark chocolate chips.

6. Pour the batter into the prepared loaf pan and bake for 25-30 minutes.

Nutritional Information:
- Calories: 180
- Protein: 6g
- Carbohydrates: 15g
- Fiber: 3g
- Potassium: 160mg

10. Baked Egg Custard

Ingredients:
- 2 cups almond milk
- 4 large eggs
- ¼ cup honey or maple syrup
- 1 teaspoon vanilla extract
- ¼ teaspoon nutmeg

Preparation:

1. Preheat oven to 325°F (163°C) and grease individual ramekins.
2. In a bowl, whisk together almond milk, eggs, honey or maple syrup, vanilla extract, and nutmeg.
3. Pour the mixture into the prepared ramekins.
4. Place ramekins in a baking dish and fill the dish with hot water.

5. Bake the custard for 30 to 35 minutes, or until it sets.

Nutritional Information:
- Calories: 120
- Protein: 6g
- Carbohydrates: 10g
- Fiber: 1g
- Potassium: 180mg

30 Day Meal Plan

Week 1

Day 1:

Breakfast: Raspberry Peach Breakfast Smoothie

Lunch: Baked Salmon with Herbed Quinoa Salad

Dinner: Nutmeg and Chicken Soup

Snack: Marinated Berries

Dessert: Chocolate Beet Cake

Day 2:

Breakfast: Egg and Veggie Muffin

Lunch: Vegetable Fish Bake

Dinner: Squash and Turmeric Soup

Snack: Veggie Snack

Dessert: Chocolate Muffins

Day 3:

Breakfast: Raspberry Overnight Porridge

Lunch: Fish and Chips with Mushy Peas

Dinner: Cabbage Turkey Soup

Snack: Spicy Crab Dip

Dessert: Pineapple Cake

Day 4:

Breakfast: Spicy Corn Bread

Lunch: Seafood Corn Chowder

Dinner: Classic Chicken Soup

Snack: Sweet and Spicy Tortilla Chips

Dessert: Strawberry Pie

Day 5:

Breakfast: Summer Veggie Omelet

Lunch: Baked Cod and Mushroom

Dinner: Mediterranean Vegetable Soup

Snack: Buffalo Chicken Dip

Dessert: Sweet Raspberry Candy

Day 6:

Breakfast: Corn Bread with Southern Twist

Lunch: Eggplant Seafood Casserole

Dinner: Oxtail Soup

Snack: Mango Chiller

Dessert: Jeweled Cookies

Day 7:

Breakfast: Breakfast Maple Sausage

Lunch: Shrimp and Pasta Salad

Dinner: Turkey and Lemongrass Soup

Snack: Vegetable Rolls

Dessert: Frozen Lemon Dessert

Week 2

Day 8:

Breakfast: Spicy Corn Bread

Lunch: Seafood Corn Chowder

Dinner: Classic Chicken Soup

Snack: Sweet and Spicy Tortilla Chips

Dessert: Strawberry Pie

Day 9:

Breakfast: Summer Veggie Omelet

Lunch: Baked Cod and Mushroom

Dinner: Mediterranean Vegetable Soup

Snack: Buffalo Chicken Dip

Dessert: Sweet Raspberry Candy

Day 10:

Breakfast: Raspberry Peach Breakfast Smoothie

Lunch: Baked Salmon with Herbed Quinoa Salad

Dinner: Nutmeg and Chicken Soup

Snack: Marinated Berries

Dessert: Chocolate Beet Cake

Day 11:

Breakfast: Corn Bread with Southern Twist

Lunch: Eggplant Seafood Casserole

Dinner: Oxtail Soup

Snack: Mango Chiller

Dessert: Jeweled Cookies

Day 12:

Breakfast: Egg and Veggie Muffin

Lunch: Vegetable Fish Bake

Dinner: Squash and Turmeric Soup

Snack: Veggie Snack

Dessert: Chocolate Muffins

Day 13:

Breakfast: Breakfast Maple Sausage

Lunch: Shrimp and Pasta Salad

Dinner: Turkey and Lemongrass Soup

Snack: Vegetable Rolls

Dessert: Frozen Lemon Dessert

Day 14:

Breakfast: Summer Veggie Omelet

Lunch: Baked Cod and Mushroom

Dinner: Mediterranean Vegetable Soup

Snack: Buffalo Chicken Dip

Dessert: Sweet Raspberry Candy

Week 3

Day 15:

Breakfast: Corn Bread with Southern Twist

Lunch: Eggplant Seafood Casserole

Dinner: Oxtail Soup

Snack: Mango Chiller

Dessert: Jeweled Cookies

Day 16:

Breakfast: Breakfast Maple Sausage

Lunch: Shrimp and Pasta Salad

Dinner: Turkey and Lemongrass Soup

Snack: Vegetable Rolls

Dessert: Frozen Lemon Dessert

Day 17:

Breakfast: Raspberry Peach Breakfast Smoothie

Lunch: Baked Salmon with Herbed Quinoa Salad

Dinner: Nutmeg and Chicken Soup

Snack: Marinated Berries

Dessert: Chocolate Beet Cake

Day 18:

Breakfast: Egg and Veggie Muffin

Lunch: Vegetable Fish Bake

Dinner: Squash and Turmeric Soup

Snack: Veggie Snack

Dessert: Chocolate Muffins

Day 19:

Breakfast: Raspberry Overnight Porridge

Lunch: Fish and Chips with Mushy Peas

Dinner: Cabbage Turkey Soup

Snack: Spicy Crab Dip

Dessert: Pineapple Cake

Day 20:

Breakfast: Spicy Corn Bread

Lunch: Seafood Corn Chowder

Dinner: Classic Chicken Soup

Snack: Sweet and Spicy Tortilla Chips

Dessert: Strawberry Pie

Day 21:

Breakfast: Summer Veggie Omelet

Lunch: Baked Cod and Mushroom

Dinner: Mediterranean Vegetable Soup

Snack: Buffalo Chicken Dip

Dessert: Sweet Raspberry Candy

Week 4

Day 22:

Breakfast: Corn Bread with Southern Twist

Lunch: Eggplant Seafood Casserole

Dinner: Oxtail Soup

Snack: Mango Chiller

Dessert: Jeweled Cookies

Day 23:

Breakfast: Breakfast Maple Sausage

Lunch: Shrimp and Pasta Salad

Dinner: Turkey and Lemongrass Soup

Snack: Vegetable Rolls

Dessert: Frozen Lemon Dessert

Day 24:

Breakfast: Raspberry Overnight Porridge

Lunch: Fish and Chips with Mushy Peas

Dinner: Cabbage Turkey Soup

Snack: Spicy Crab Dip

Dessert: Pineapple Cake

Day 25:

Breakfast: Spicy Corn Bread

Lunch: Seafood Corn Chowder

Dinner: Classic Chicken Soup

Snack: Sweet and Spicy Tortilla Chips

Dessert: Strawberry Pie

Day 26:

Breakfast: Summer Veggie Omelet

Lunch: Baked Cod and Mushroom

Dinner: Mediterranean Vegetable Soup

Snack: Buffalo Chicken Dip

Dessert: Sweet Raspberry Candy

Day 27:

Breakfast: Raspberry Peach Breakfast Smoothie

Lunch: Baked Salmon with Herbed Quinoa Salad

Dinner: Nutmeg and Chicken Soup

Snack: Marinated Berries

Dessert: Chocolate Beet Cake

Day 28:

Breakfast: Egg and Veggie Muffin

Lunch: Vegetable Fish Bake

Dinner: Squash and Turmeric Soup

Snack: Veggie Snack

Dessert: Chocolate Muffins

Day 29:

Breakfast: Breakfast Maple Sausage

Lunch: Shrimp and Pasta Salad

Dinner: Turkey and Lemongrass Soup

Snack: Vegetable Rolls

Dessert: Frozen Lemon Dessert

Day 30:

Breakfast: Raspberry Overnight Porridge

Lunch: Fish and Chips with Mushy Peas

Dinner: Cabbage Turkey Soup

Snack: Spicy Crab Dip

Dessert: Pineapple Cake

CONCLUSION

I'd like to end by sincerely thanking you for starting your path toward improved health by following the Kidney Disease Diet for Seniors on Stage 3. I respect your faith in this extensive guide and your dedication to learning about and adopting a kidney-friendly lifestyle.

I genuinely hope you find happiness and fulfillment in every nourishing bite as you delve into the many and delectable dishes customized for your particular need. It can be difficult to follow a diet for renal disease, but your commitment to your health is an inspiration of your fortitude and resilience.

I hope you have vibrant health, a resurgence of energy, and the peace of mind that comes from making wise decisions for your body. I hope this book is a useful tool for you as you work to improve your kidney health and that each dish helps you get closer to living the healthy, active life you deserve.

Keep in mind that taking care of your health now will pay off in the future by making positive changes to your life. I wish you good health and hope that this book turns out to be the answer you've been looking for to reach the best possible kidney health.

My Little Request

Dear Reader,

Thanks for your purchase, hope you enjoyed reading.

Could you please take a few seconds to leave a positive feedback on this book?

It'll help reach more people and we can collectively help reverse this deadly disease.

Thank you.

BONUS: WEEKLY MEAL PLANNER JOURNAL

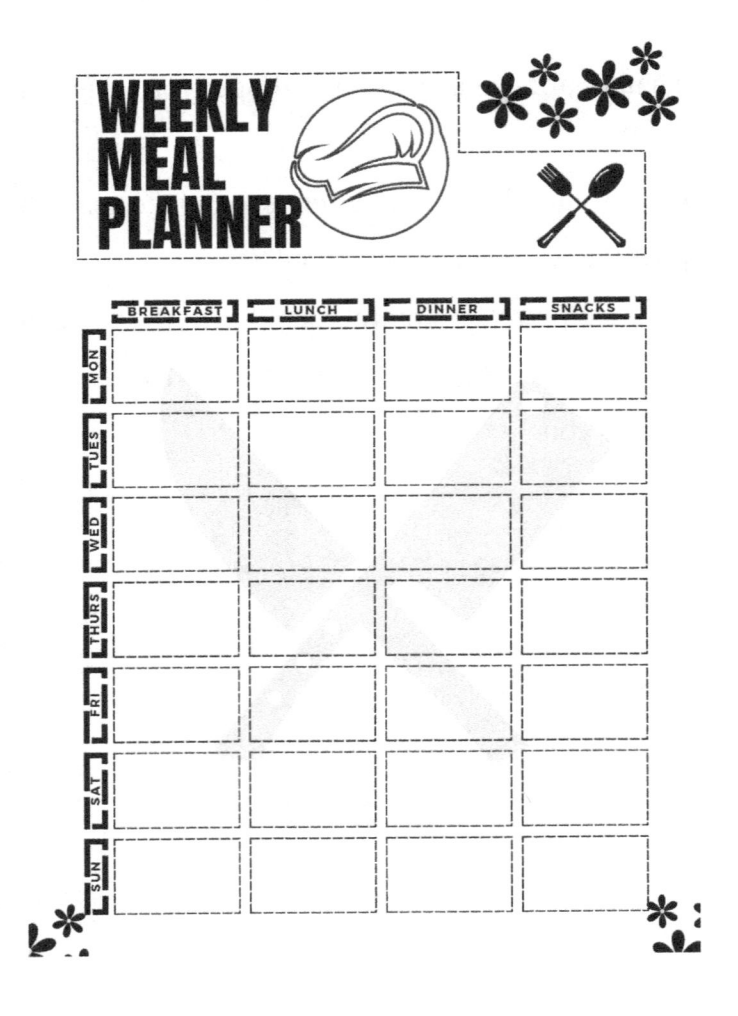

WEEKLY MEAL PLANNER

	BREAKFAST	LUNCH	DINNER	SNACKS
MON				
TUES				
WED				
THURS				
FRI				
SAT				
SUN				

WEEKLY MEAL PLANNER

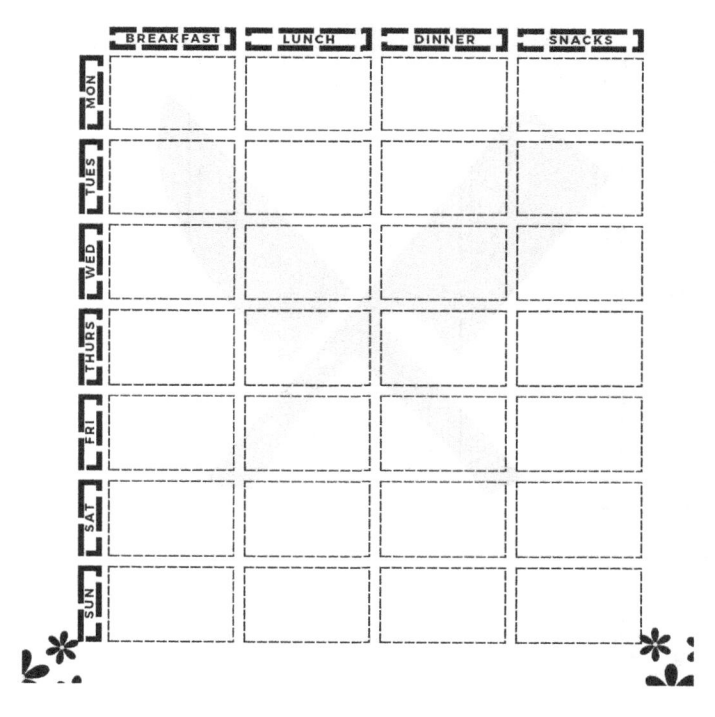

	BREAKFAST	LUNCH	DINNER	SNACKS
MON				
TUES				
WED				
THURS				
FRI				
SAT				
SUN				

WEEKLY MEAL PLANNER

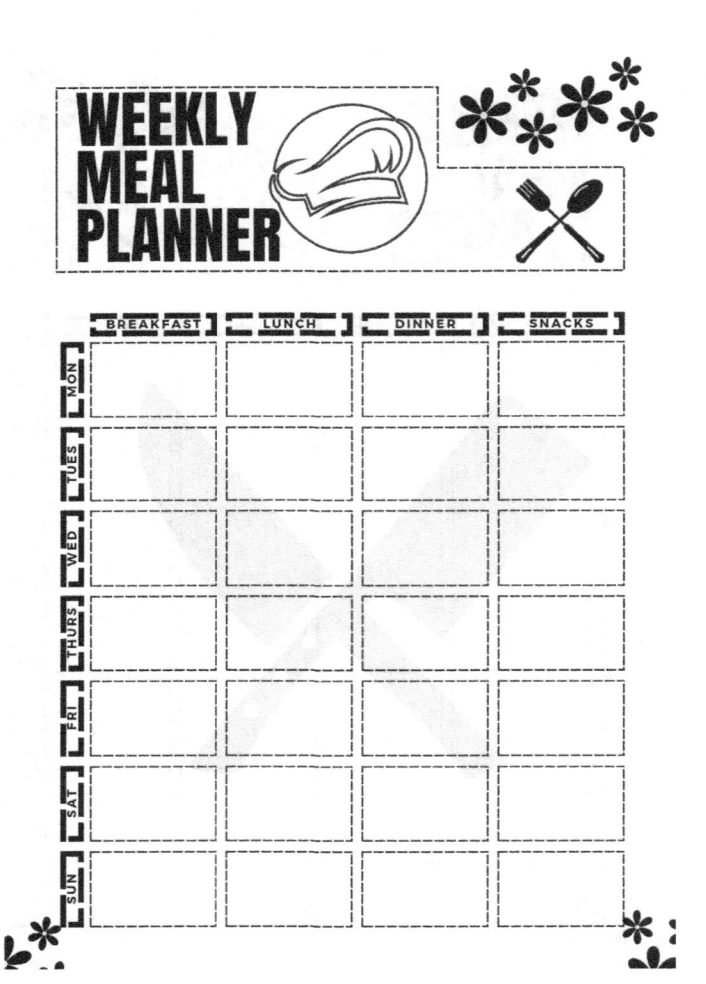

	BREAKFAST	LUNCH	DINNER	SNACKS
MON				
TUES				
WED				
THURS				
FRI				
SAT				
SUN				

WEEKLY MEAL PLANNER

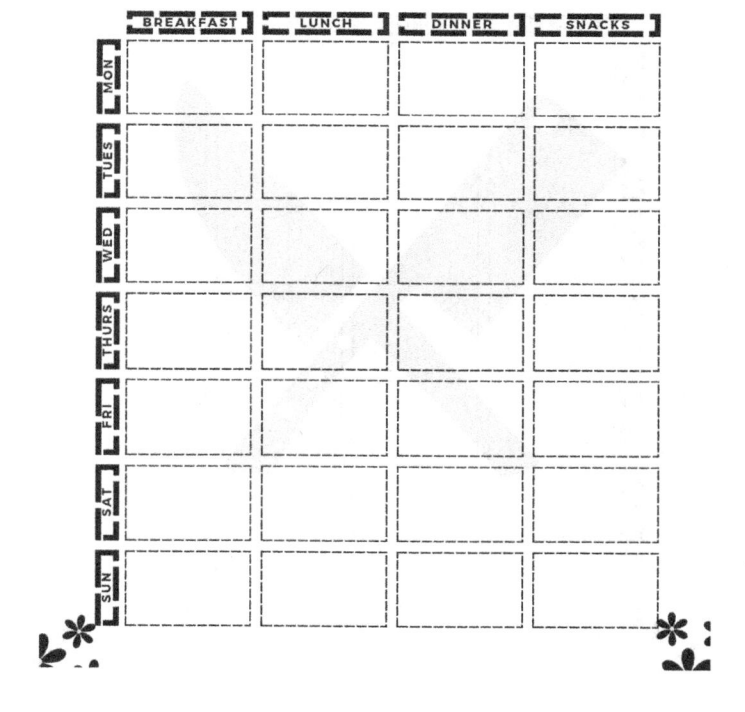

	BREAKFAST	LUNCH	DINNER	SNACKS
MON				
TUES				
WED				
THURS				
FRI				
SAT				
SUN				

KIDNEY DISEASE DIET FOR SENIORS ON STAGE 3

WEEKLY MEAL PLANNER

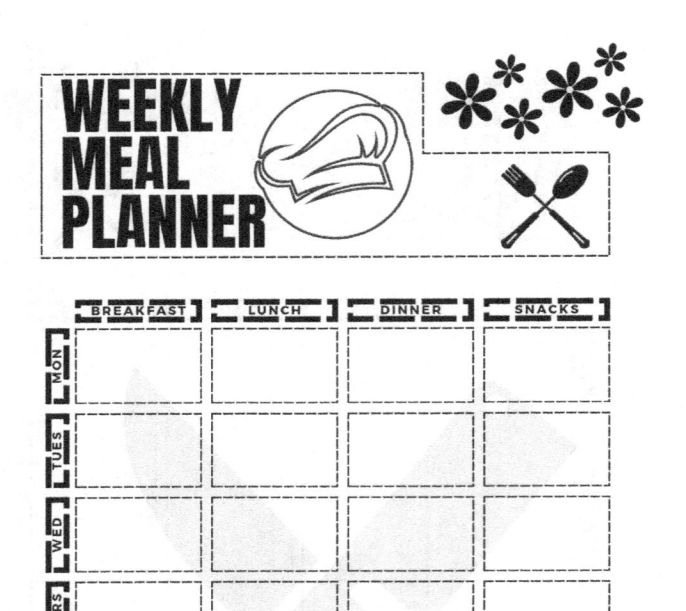

	BREAKFAST	LUNCH	DINNER	SNACKS
MON				
TUES				
WED				
THURS				
FRI				
SAT				
SUN				

KIDNEY DISEASE DIET FOR SENIORS ON STAGE 3

WEEKLY MEAL PLANNER

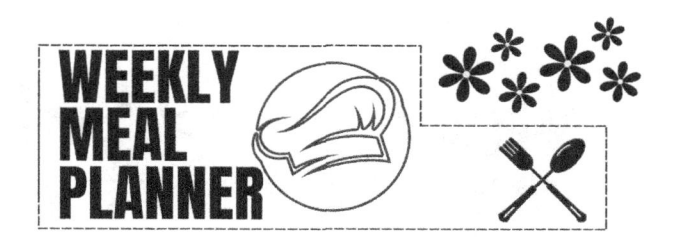

	BREAKFAST	LUNCH	DINNER	SNACKS
MON				
TUES				
WED				
THURS				
FRI				
SAT				
SUN				

WEEKLY MEAL PLANNER

	BREAKFAST	LUNCH	DINNER	SNACKS
MON				
TUES				
WED				
THURS				
FRI				
SAT				
SUN				

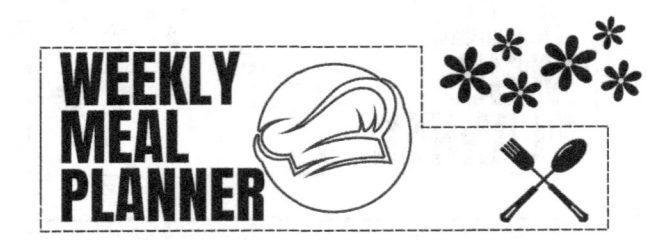

WEEKLY MEAL PLANNER

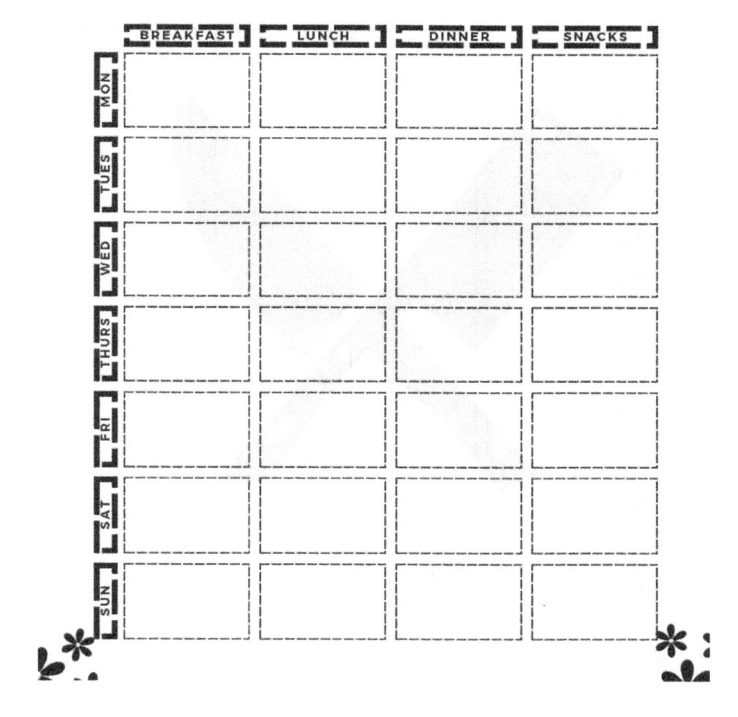

	BREAKFAST	LUNCH	DINNER	SNACKS
MON				
TUES				
WED				
THURS				
FRI				
SAT				
SUN				

WEEKLY MEAL PLANNER

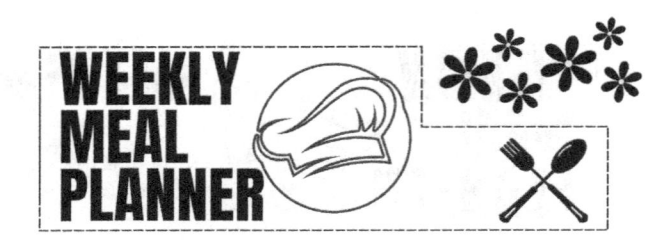

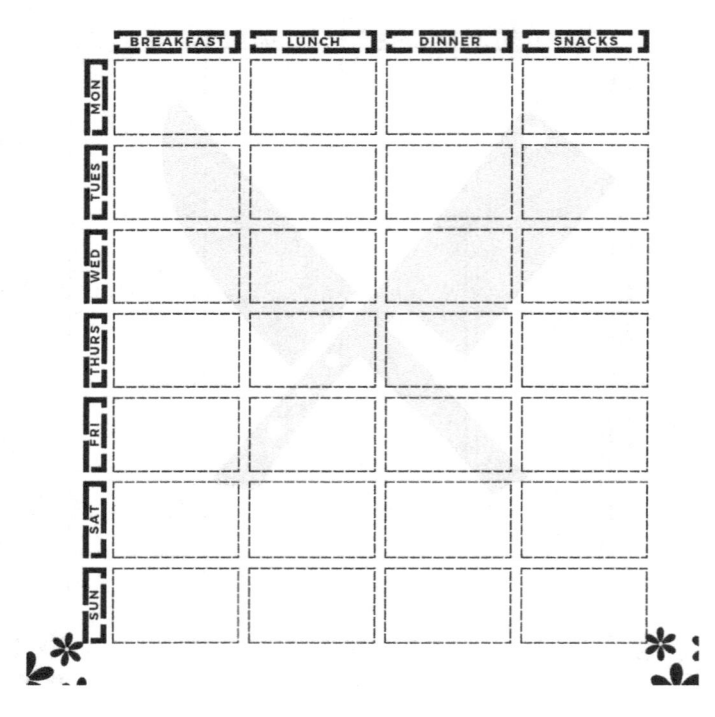

	BREAKFAST	LUNCH	DINNER	SNACKS
MON				
TUES				
WED				
THURS				
FRI				
SAT				
SUN				

KIDNEY DISEASE DIET FOR SENIORS ON STAGE 3

WEEKLY MEAL PLANNER

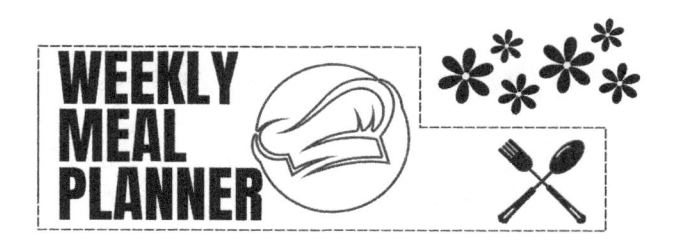

	BREAKFAST	LUNCH	DINNER	SNACKS
MON				
TUES				
WED				
THURS				
FRI				
SAT				
SUN				

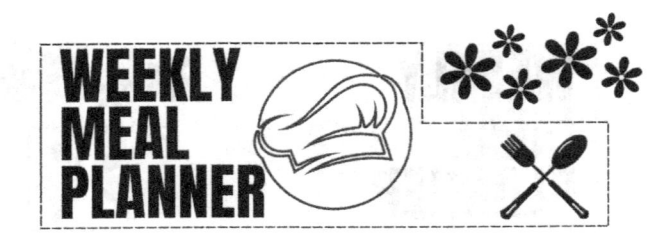

Weekly Meal Planner

	BREAKFAST	LUNCH	DINNER	SNACKS
MON				
TUES				
WED				
THURS				
FRI				
SAT				
SUN				

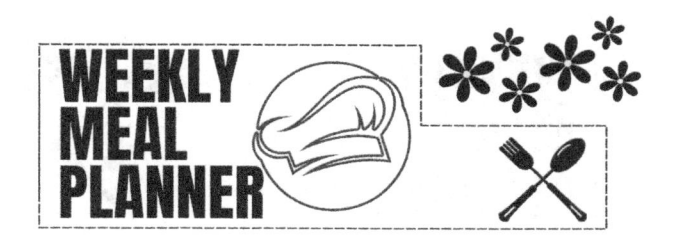

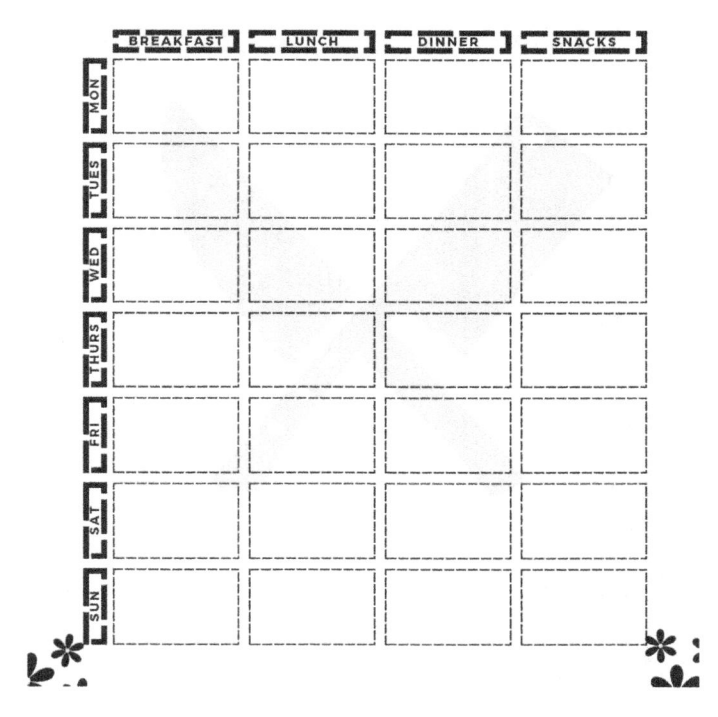

WEEKLY MEAL PLANNER

	BREAKFAST	LUNCH	DINNER	SNACKS
MON				
TUES				
WED				
THURS				
FRI				
SAT				
SUN				

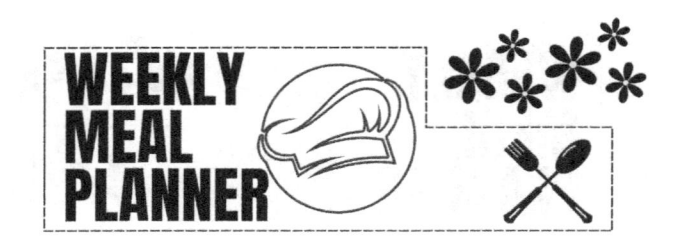

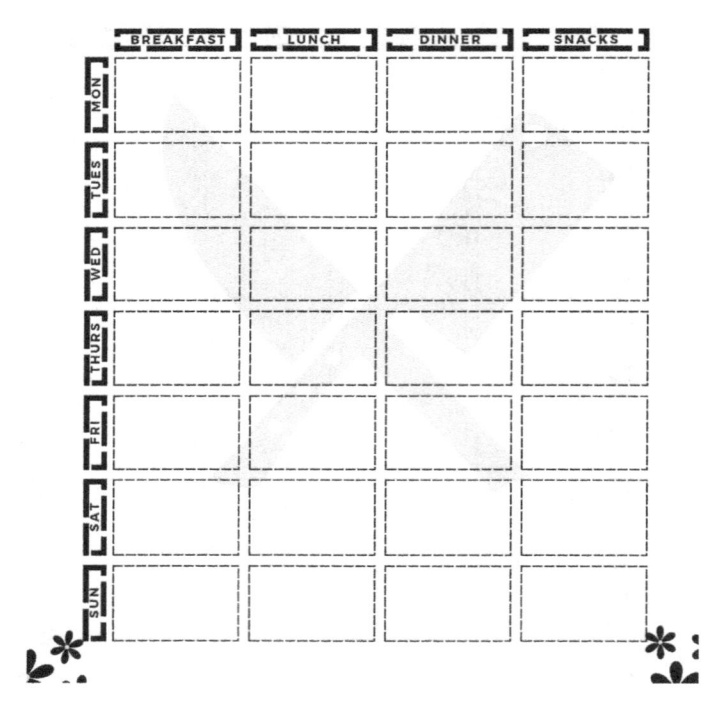

WEEKLY MEAL PLANNER

	BREAKFAST	LUNCH	DINNER	SNACKS
MON				
TUES				
WED				
THURS				
FRI				
SAT				
SUN				

WEEKLY MEAL PLANNER

	BREAKFAST	LUNCH	DINNER	SNACKS
MON				
TUES				
WED				
THURS				
FRI				
SAT				
SUN				

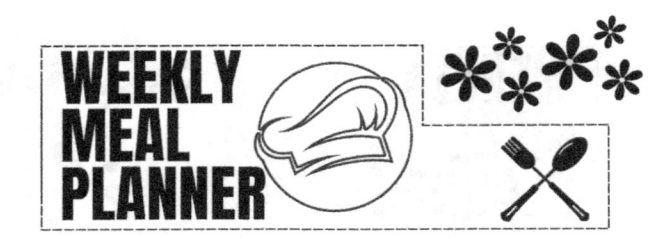

WEEKLY MEAL PLANNER

	BREAKFAST	LUNCH	DINNER	SNACKS
MON				
TUES				
WED				
THURS				
FRI				
SAT				
SUN				

WEEKLY MEAL PLANNER

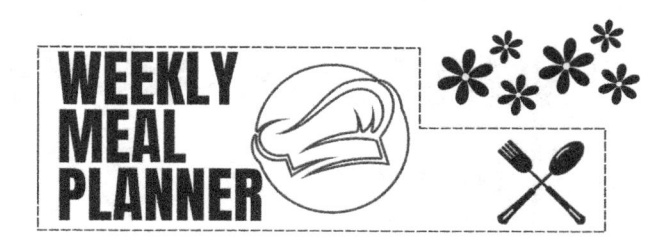

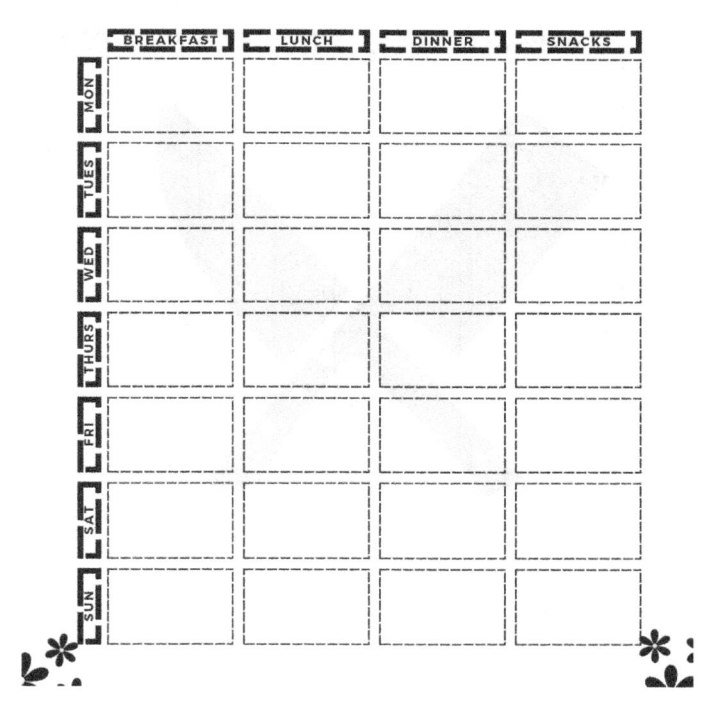

	BREAKFAST	LUNCH	DINNER	SNACKS
MON				
TUES				
WED				
THURS				
FRI				
SAT				
SUN				

WEEKLY MEAL PLANNER

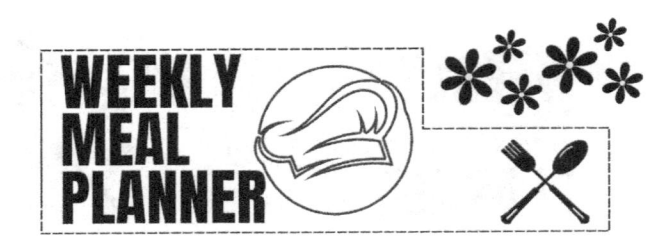

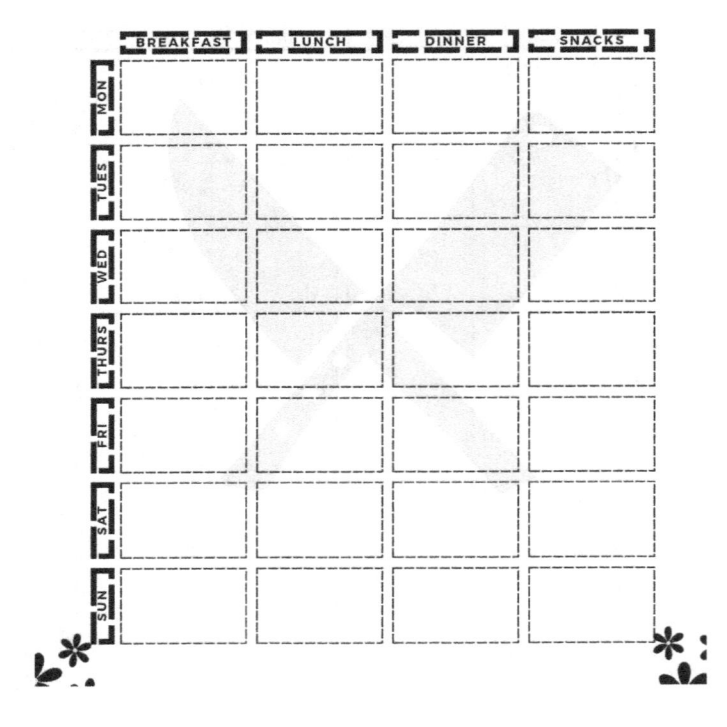

	BREAKFAST	LUNCH	DINNER	SNACKS
MON				
TUES				
WED				
THURS				
FRI				
SAT				
SUN				

KIDNEY DISEASE DIET FOR SENIORS ON STAGE 3

WEEKLY MEAL PLANNER

	BREAKFAST	LUNCH	DINNER	SNACKS
MON				
TUES				
WED				
THURS				
FRI				
SAT				
SUN				

WEEKLY MEAL PLANNER

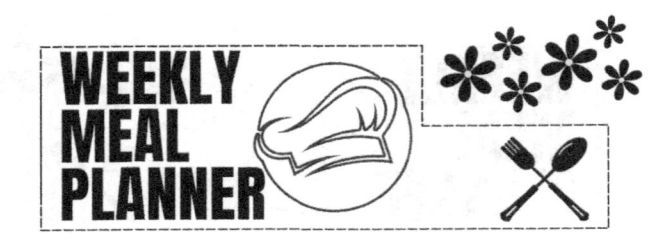

	BREAKFAST	LUNCH	DINNER	SNACKS
MON				
TUES				
WED				
THURS				
FRI				
SAT				
SUN				

WEEKLY MEAL PLANNER

	BREAKFAST	LUNCH	DINNER	SNACKS
MON				
TUES				
WED				
THURS				
FRI				
SAT				
SUN				

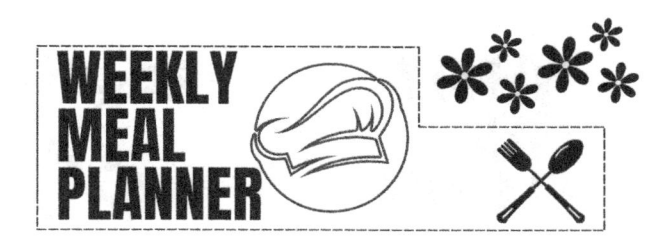

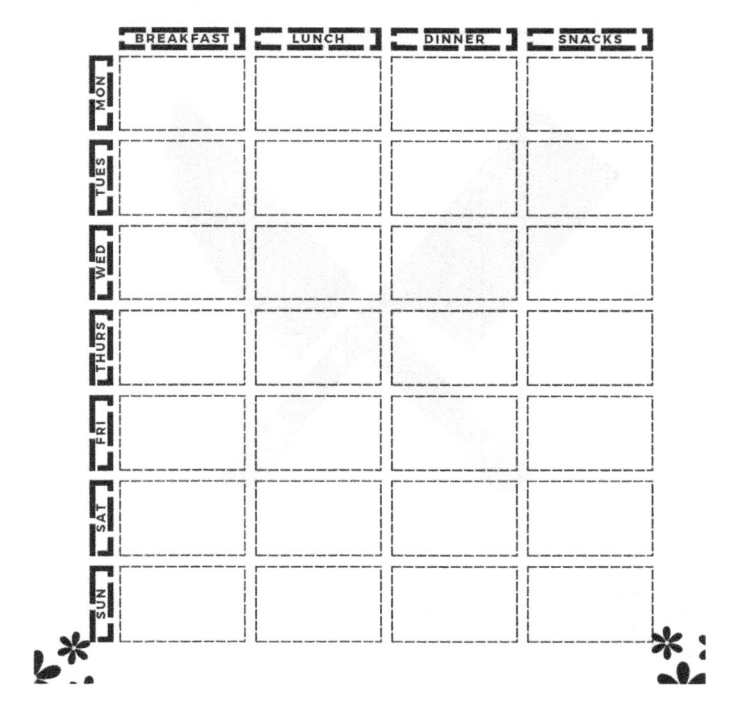

WEEKLY MEAL PLANNER

	BREAKFAST	LUNCH	DINNER	SNACKS
MON				
TUES				
WED				
THURS				
FRI				
SAT				
SUN				

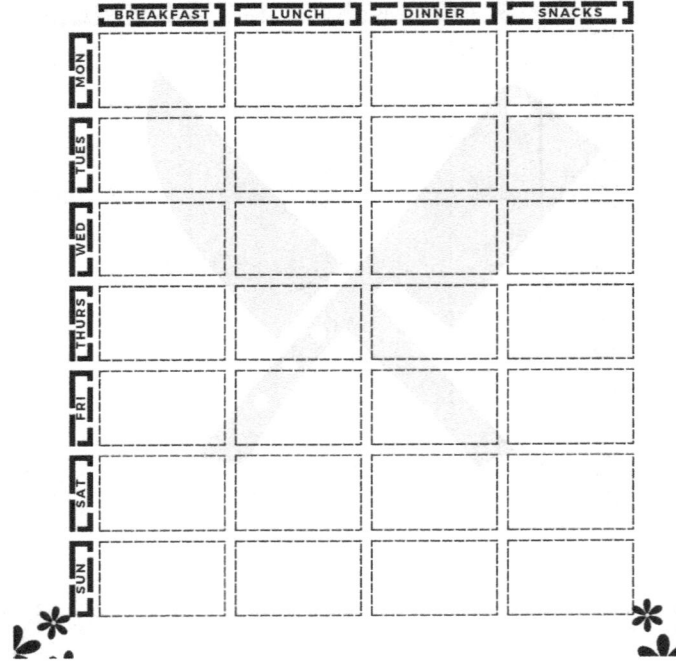

KIDNEY DISEASE DIET FOR SENIORS ON STAGE 3

WEEKLY MEAL PLANNER

	BREAKFAST	LUNCH	DINNER	SNACKS
MON				
TUES				
WED				
THURS				
FRI				
SAT				
SUN				

WEEKLY MEAL PLANNER

	BREAKFAST	LUNCH	DINNER	SNACKS
MON				
TUES				
WED				
THURS				
FRI				
SAT				
SUN				

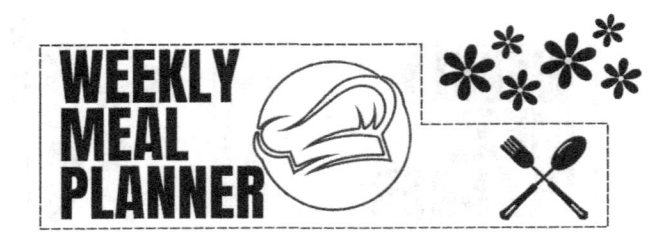

WEEKLY MEAL PLANNER

	BREAKFAST	LUNCH	DINNER	SNACKS
MON				
TUES				
WED				
THURS				
FRI				
SAT				
SUN				

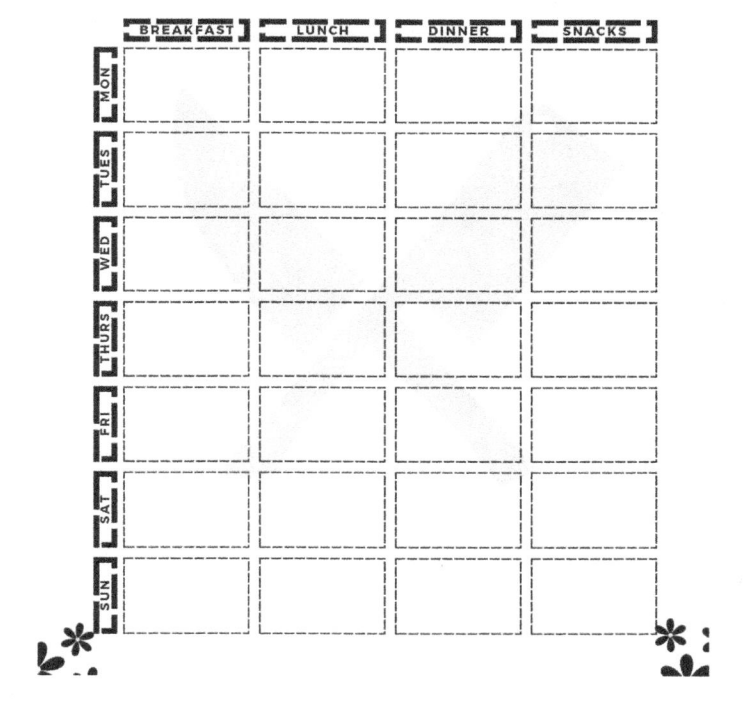

Made in United States
North Haven, CT
03 July 2024